FOR
REGISTERED
NURSES
IN
INPATIENT CARE

NURSING NARRATIVE NOTE EXAMPLES

to Save Your License

UPDATED 2nd EDITION

LENA EMPYEMA

Nursing Narrative Note Examples
to Save Your License

for Registered Nurses in Inpatient Care

UPDATED 2ND EDITION

Lena Empyema
by ZEPHRY™

What You'll Learn Inside

- When to use a narrative note
- Components of an effective narrative note
- How to refer to yourself and others
- How to phrase your notes
- The best practice for referring to time
- Common phrases to avoid
- About double documentation
- HIPAA specific to narrative notes
- Abbreviations
- Tips to streamline your narrative note writing process
- The notes to write for every patient on every shift
- 44 specific examples for situations commonly encountered in medical/surgical or lower acuity units

44 Examples Inside

- Assumption of care
- Provider at bedside
- End of shift handoff
- New admission
- Admit from emergency department
- Admit from PACU
- Admit from clinic
- Inventory of belongings on admission
- General surgery pre-op
- General surgery post op
- S/p bariatric surgery
- S/p gynecologic surgery
- Patient transport off ward
- Ambulation
- IV initiation
- Venipuncture
- Foley placement
- NG insertion
- S/p TKA
- S/p THA
- S/p TSA
- Circulation assessment in surgical extremity
- Physical therapy consult
- Occupational therapy consult
- Gynecological diagnosis
- Urological diagnosis
- Gastrointestinal diagnosis
- High risk for falls
- IV infiltration
- Allergic reaction
- Blood product reaction
- Fall without injury

- Fall with injury
- Follow up after a fall
- Leaving AMA
- Non-compliance with provider's orders on diet restriction
- Refusing medication
- New onset arrhythmia, asymptomatic
- New onset arrythmia, symptomatic,
- Equipment malfunction
- Naloxone for overdose
- Rapid response
- Code blue
- Discharge
- Transfer to outside facility

About the Author

I'm Lena Empyema, the author of this book, and also an RN-MSN with more than 10 years spent working in healthcare. I choose to write under this pen name that's easier to spell and remember than my own last name, so while the moniker is an alias, my credential are real. I have found a passion for empowering fellow nurses by providing education about charting and documentation, an area where my co-workers and I historically had endless questions with ambiguous answers. I didn't start my nursing career expecting to become a subject matter expert on nurse documentation, but after completing a thesis for my Master's in Nursing Science degree on the topic of charting and subsequently continuing in-depth research on it for years afterward, here is where I found myself. Now, empowering nurses through education is my passion!

I have published multiple resources with the goal of helping nurses take charge of their shifts and their careers. In 2021, I founded my new business **Zephry** at www.zephryco.com to offer my unique **QuickBrain™ Reusable Nurse Report** notebook to streamline the report process and make it easy to track the ever-changing information that nurses need to keep straight for up to 12 hours, and also my own **working template** for notes that you can download and start implementing in your own charting right away.

I'm not an attorney and this is not legal advice. This book is all of the information I have compiled as a result of years of research to bring clarity to those gray areas my colleagues and I struggled with when trying to document our shifts.

-Lena Empyema

Narrative Notes & When to Use Them

Chapter Overview:

- **Narrative notes help nurses tell the whole story.**
- **Notes help you defend your actions.**
- **Writing narrative notes can be a quick, informal process.**

In the age of electronic medical records, drop-down boxes and fill-in-the-blanks replace many free-texted notes. Plugging values into the EMR is faster for the nurse, and is more efficient for other health care providers or auditors to review certain data points. However, they don't always tell the whole story. Understanding that the purpose of documentation is, in fact, to ensure that every pertinent aspect of a patient's status and care during a particular shift is captured, it can sometimes be necessary to write notes to supplement the data in flowsheets to ensure that all necessary information is captured.

This is especially true when things don't go according to plan. Adverse events, quotes from patients that could affect a provider's decisions about the patient's plan of care, and deviations from prescribed orders (whether due to a safety issue or the patient's noncompliance) are best captured in free-texted notes.

Other purposes for narrative notes include documented proof that you performed a certain intervention within your scope of practice and while keeping the patient safe. For example, if you transport a patient from a room on the third floor to the first floor for an x-ray, there may not be a drop-down box option in the medical record for you to specify that you used a portable oxygen tank to continue delivering 4 lpm of oxygen via a nasal cannula during the transport for your patient with COPD. It may seem like common sense that you made sure your oxygen-dependent patient had oxygen available during the half hour that she spent in imaging. But, what if it's not documented in the patient's chart that she had oxygen available during her transport? What if she encounters respiratory distress an hour after she gets back to the floor, and the rapid response team can't find any proof that she was receiving oxygen therapy during an extended period of time, and it becomes your word against someone else's? Taking thirty seconds to write a narrative note specifying that you ensured the patient had a portable oxygen tank with her could save you from questions and stress later.

If you just scoffed because there's no way you can finish a note in thirty seconds, not that you would have thirty spare seconds in the middle of your shift anyway, I have good news. It really can be that quick. Writing a narrative note doesn't have to be a lengthy process requiring thought and planning. In fact, I dug deep into the topic during my research to determine the best way to phrase vital information in narrative notes, and it turns out that the preferred format is also the least wordy and the fastest to type. I'll elaborate on that in a few more sections.

To put it simply, a narrative note should be written any time adequate information in the flowsheet of the EMR doesn't tell the complete picture. Whether prompted by a supervisor or not, whether the most seasoned nurse twenty years your senior recommends it or not, a narrative note should supplement the information captured elsewhere in the chart with a quick blurb that completes the story. Doing so can help you defend your decisions in the future and has the potential to save your license.

Components of an Effective Note

Chapter Overview

- **Phrase narrative notes in blurbs that omit pronouns.**
- **HIPAA regulations don't include names of staff members.**
- **Don't speculate or dig for answers you don't have.**

Now that you know when to write a narrative note, how should you format it? In short, there is not a specific black and white format for writing a narrative note. Even the Joint Commission specifies that the exact format of nursing documentation is not something they mandate. Rather, the Joint Commission is simply concerned with the content that is documented in a patient chart, no matter where or how it is in there.

Since working as a nurse is mostly about learning and adhering to very specific policies and procedures in a textbook way, it can feel like a weight taken off to know that memorizing a certain format for narrative notes isn't something you'll have to do. However, the gray area can lead to uncertainty about whether a note is sufficient to defend your actions at a later time. It can make the process more difficult when you sit down at a computer, a running to-do list of twenty other tasks at the forefront of your mind, fingers hovering over the keyboard, and you're stricken with writer's block. *How do I explain what just happened?*

While the usual places nurses look for guidance, such as the state nurse practice acts and the Joint Commission's resources, don't specify how to write a note or what to say, I spent hours reaching out to legal nurse consultants and malpractice attorneys to pick their brains and determine what formatting and phrasing they have found effective when reviewing their countless charts for court cases.

FORMAT

Through my career, I have found a general belief among nurses that narrative notes must be penned in the third person. When I was a new nurse, I was coached by the more seasoned staff that all narrative notes should be phrased "this nurse witnessed a fall. This nurse activated the emergency response system." It's awkward to write like that, and it's awkward to read. And there's no point.

I specifically asked malpractice attorneys who read hundreds of charts if there is a real reason that first person point of view cannot be used in narrative notes. I wanted to know why I couldn't just write more fluidly, such as "I witnessed a fall. I then activated the emergency response system." As it turned out, the aversion to first person in nurse notes has just inexplicably become the culture.

I dug further, though, not yet confident enough to tell all my colleagues, "It's okay, just write narrative notes the same way you'd write an email to your supervisor!" While I wasn't able to find concrete data dictating the point of view of nursing narrative notes, I did find more specific guidelines for the notes written by physicians. That research revealed that physicians are instructed to simply omit pronouns altogether when they write their notes.

If you've read many History & Physical notes, SOAP notes, or progress notes written by providers, you've likely seen the same broad range of formatting and phrasing that I've seen. Not every physician writes to exclude pronouns. But, some do. And reading a note written in incomplete sentences, I found, is actually faster and easier to read. It gets straight to the point. There's no confusion about who the provider is referring to in the note, because I know that if the note appears in a patient's chart, the note is about that patient. I know that if the electronic stamp states that Dr. Smith wrote that note, then Dr. Smith wrote that note.

Another benefit to writing a note in incomplete sentences without pronouns is that it's faster. It's a lot faster. It helps you omit all of the fluff, get straight to the point, and get on with your shift.

So, rather than writing your notes in first person like you would an email, my guidance for narrative notes is to write as if you're texting a friend a complete story: short blurbs, periods after every thought, no use of pronouns, no awkward third-person references.

CONTENT

With the formatting established, what about the content? What information is truly pertinent in a narrative note, and what should not be included?

As I stated, a narrative note should help you tell a complete story. It should fill in the blanks of the patient's chart where there may not be sufficient values and data in the flowsheets and drop-down boxes for someone externally reviewing it to truly tell the whole story of what happened.

What if part of your story is told elsewhere in the chart? For example, what if you're narrating the events that took place after the patient fall I referenced earlier? You (hopefully) have multiple sets of vital signs. You probably asked the patient about pain. You likely asked the patient what he or she had been doing that led to the fall.

The vital signs should then be entered in their normal place in the EMR, likely on a flowsheet. After the vital signs are entered into that flowsheet, that part of the story is told. It's done, and you don't need to write the vital signs again in your note. Actually, doing so creates room for errors and confusion. Any time you double document information, you run into the risk of creating a discrepancy. It could look like you may have taken two sets of vital signs that were exactly the same. Worse, you could fail to transcribe one of the sets of data identically, creating even more confusion. You don't need to put values in more than one place in the chart. For this specific example, in your narrative note, you can then simply state, "see vital sign flow sheet."

What if another nurse got to your patient's room at the same time as you to witness the patient lying on the floor, and that nurse says, "I'll write the narrative note. You have enough going on."

That kind of teamwork and support is invaluable! It was very nice of your colleague to offer to document the event so you can take care of notifying the physician, likely transporting the patient to imaging for a CT scan, et cetera. However, delegating the entirety of documentation to a willing colleague is not something you should do. The other nurse to witness the fall should certainly write a quick note, stating exactly what happened from her point of view. However, that note should not take the place of yours. If a patient assigned to your care experiences a sentinel event, you should always write a note stating the facts from your point of view.

It's okay to check with your co-workers about the events that occurred before writing your note. Doing so is not nefarious-you're not murder suspects attempting to "get your stories straight" before being questioned by the police. Rather, your head is probably in six different places at once. When things go wrong, they do so quickly, and if you blink, you could miss an important piece of the story. Perhaps you witnessed your patient fall, and from your point of view, it appeared to happen out of nowhere. You're flustered and you can't even remember if your patient fell on her left or her right side. But your co-worker in the doorway reminded you that the patient fell onto her knees and caught her fall with her right hand. "Remember, she had her right hand on the floor still when you stooped down to support her left arm and ask if she was okay?" With the help of your colleague, you do remember that.

What you cannot do is get pieces of the story from other witnesses if you truly did not see with your own eyes. Doing so is called hearsay, and it shouldn't be included in your narrative notes. Hearsay, in this example, could be including a line in your note, "Samantha saw the patient trip over a pair of slippers." Your narrative notes shouldn't be used to put words in other people's mouths, or claim something to be true that you did not witness with your own eyes.

Along the same lines, you should not speculate as to causation of certain events if you are not sure what precipitated something to occur. Nurses tend to think like scientists. We like to understand why things are happening. Our brains tend to dwell on the evidence and subconsciously consider plausible scenarios. It's okay to speculate with colleagues during debriefing, such as, "she had just finished that entire mug of water. I'll bet she had to pee so badly she was rushing to the bathroom and she ended up falling." But concrete facts that you witnessed yourself are the only things that should appear in the narrative notes that you write.

Similarly, keep all of the information objective. Narrative notes are not the right place to express opinions about a patient's plan of care, nor to pass judgement. Nurses are all human, and we work in environments that can be heavily emotionally charged. If you feel subjective thoughts clouding your ability to write a completely objective narrative note, take five minutes to focus yourself on another task before coming back to finish the note with only the facts. Your professional license and your career are not worth whatever you may think you're accomplishing with passive aggression or opinionated statements in a patient chart.

LENGTH

How long should a narrative note be? However long it takes to tell the story. The proper length for a note truly isn't defined. Understanding that most narrative notes are for the purpose of explaining what happened and what you did about it, it would be difficult to write an adequate narrative note in fewer than two blurbs. Each blurb can be an incomplete sentence as discussed, but each separate thought should still be separated by a period.

On the opposite end of the spectrum, it is also possible to be too wordy in a narrative note. Again, perhaps frustratingly, there is not a specific length that would be generally considered "too long." In my prior practice, I have written narrative notes that easily would fill an entire page in a Word document describing a complex sentinel event that occurred requiring a great deal of intervention before a satisfactory conclusion was made.

If you follow the guideline of writing straight to the point to explain what happened, how you reacted, and the overall outcome using the short phrasing with pronouns omitted from sentences, you are most likely to write a note of an appropriate length.

Keep in mind also that if two nurses were asked to write about the same event that they each witnessed, the nurses may draft notes of two different lengths, and it doesn't mean either of them is wrong or inadequate.

Rather than focusing on a certain length, focus instead on the quality of the content and ensuring that the right questions are answered.

Concept of Time Within Notes

Chapter Overview:

- **Use a 24-hour time format when possible.**
- **Understand that every note you write has an electronic time stamp attached.**
- **Complete charting within 24 hours whenever possible.**

Specific Times *versus* Approximated Times

Using a 24-hour time format ("military time") is the best way to differentiate between morning and night. Most charting systems default to 24-hour time, but some still use A.M. and P.M. If yours relies on A.M. and P.M., ensure that it's easy to tell whether you're referring to a time in the morning or a time in the evening.

When you know the exact time that something occurred, specify the time in your note. But if there is a question as to exactly what time something happened, preface the time with "at approximately." For example, if you entered the patient's room at 0802 and started scanning medications into the MAR before the patient climbed out of bed and fell, you can state "entered room at 0802. Approximately two to three minutes later, patient climbed out of bed and fell to floor."

In code situations, the exact times should be known for most of the interventions performed during resuscitation efforts. There may be approximate times for when the patient was initially discovered and when CPR was first initiated, but as the code team assembles, a designated recorder should be among those present. The recorder should write down the exact times for each medication given, shock delivered, et cetera. This is an example of a time when it would be most appropriate to obtain a copy of the notes the recorder kept in order to write your narrative note with the exact times.

Electronic Timestamps

On the topic of time, your narrative notes will be time-stamped with the exact time that they are written. If you work with an EMR that allows you to change the time that the note appears to have been saved, *don't do it*. Do not alter the time attached to the note. Rather, in the note itself, designate the note a "late entry" and include only accurate times in your text.

Why? EMRs capture every timestamp. You cannot see each timestamp, but should the chart ever go under scrutinous review, there are ways to extract data beyond what you can see on your screen. Attempting to alter the time on a narrative note to make it appear as though it was written in a timelier manner can have only negative consequences. Late entries are permissible in a patient chart within a certain window of time. Attempting to skew the appearance of your documentation, on the other hand, can be considered fraudulent and can affect your credibility, especially if compiled with other findings.

What constitutes a late entry?

The short answer is that it can vary per hospital policy. Reasonably, you have the duration of your shift to complete applicable documentation in a patient chart without having to designate the entry as late. As you know, it would be a rare shift that every component of documentation is captured in real time, no matter how much hospital administration encourages it.

Some hospitals have their own policies that all charting must be completed in a mandated window. Usually, hospitals want charting to be complete within 24 hours of when the event occurred, or within 24 hours of patient discharge. Independent of hospital policies, Medicare advises that late entries can be added to a chart up to 48 hours after an event, but states that it should not be common practice to add entries to charts so late.

As a general rule, if adding data to a patient chart after your shift ends but before the 24 hour guideline has passed, simply begin the narrative note with "late entry." Then the remainder of your note should be the same as it would have been if you charted it in real time.

Pitfalls to Avoid

Chapter Overview:

- **Avoid double documentation.**
- **Don't state, "will continue to monitor."**
- **Adhere to HIPAA standards.**

Double Documentation

Double documentation is a single piece of data charted in two different places in a single chart. Triple documentation exists also, and refers to a single piece of data charted in three places.

What if your hospital's documentation policy is such that double documentation is unavoidable?

I've been in similar situations where the nurses were asked to chart a certain value in one flowsheet where the providers wanted to access it most easily, but it also needed to appear in a different part of the chart for coding and billing purposes, and sometimes, we just weren't sure that we were really covering all our bases, so we'd plug the values into our narrative notes just to make sure that there weren't any questions as to what we had done and what our outcomes were. There are probably a lot of charts floating around out there that include double and triple documentation that I entered thinking I was doing the right thing. I've learned better charting practices since then, so now I can do better.

In my experience, a hospital's administrative team does not seek to make things more difficult purposely or out of spite. I suggest initiating a conversation with your manager or supervisor, whoever feels more accessible, to discuss what you've learned in this book. You could ask about the process to revise a policy that requires double or triple documentation, citing the fact that not only will staff nurses be more protected if a chart is audited, but also that streamlining the contents of a chart helps protect the hospital as well. Further, wasting time charting data in multiple places adds to the mental workload of already overtaxed nurses.

What if you need to record a value (such as vital signs) in a single box on a flowsheet, but it requires more explanation in a narrative note?

This is a common occurrence. Rather than recording the vital sign (as an example) in the vitals flow sheet and again listing the vitals in the narrative note, refer the reader back to the flowsheet in the narrative. An example would be, "patient states she feels dizzy. Immediately obtained vital signs. See vitals flow sheet for data."

What if double documenting is absolutely, positively unavoidable?

I know I can't address every single contingency you may face on your particular unit. If you truly cannot avoid double documenting, you must ensure that the data is all exactly the same. The times should be identical, the values themselves must be identical, and there should be no discrepancies that could lead to confusion.

Stating, "will continue to monitor."

The importance of ending most notes with this tagline was drilled into me at multiple places of employment by my more senior colleagues. They had good intentions, but their recommendation to wrap up most of my notes with a promise to continue doing my job isn't actually a best practice. On the contrary, including the statement that you will continue to perform a standard aspect of your job can have negative implications.

In many hospitals, hourly rounding is the minimum standard as it is. Sometimes, rounding every two hours overnight is acceptable to facilitate sleep for stable patients. If you are rounding hourly on every patient anyway and documenting your rounds in another flow sheet, why would you need to specify again in a note on a particular patient that you will continue to do so?

Creating a pattern in your charts of specifying that you are, indeed, regularly checking in for some patients in some situations, but not for others, creates ambiguity. As I said, I've done it myself. I thought those four extra words at the end of my notes made it look like I was on top of things. Actually, all it does is create a question in my charting. Imagine a malpractice attorney poring over your charts from two years ago, wondering aloud, "If she didn't write in a note that she was monitoring other patients, was she monitoring them? It was supposed to be hospital policy to monitor her patients every hour… but she only wrote that she was continuing to monitor some patients, in some notes. What about when all she did was check a box next to 'hourly rounds?' Was she doing her job, or wasn't she?"

You have a legal obligation to tend to the patients in your care, and your hospital mandates the manner in which you should be doing so. As long as you are documenting hourly rounds per your hospital facility, you shouldn't be ending routine narrative notes with "will continue to monitor." Monitoring patients is your job when you're on shift. Don't create ambiguity in your charts by adding extra statements. Keep your narrative notes factual and centered around, **"here's what happened, here's what I did, here was the outcome."** Just as you should not try to speculate as to causation for sentinel events or include opinions or judgment in notes, don't state what you will be doing in the future, especially if it should be a core aspect of the duties on your shift anyway.

HIPAA Violations

HIPAA always applies to the nursing process, including within narrative notes. You cannot include the names of roommates or other identifying patient information for anyone other than the patient on whom you are charting.

As a quick refresher, not because you're not already drilled on HIPAA compliance within your hospital system, but because HIPAA is generally not discussed in this context: names of hospital employees such as nurses and physicians are not protected by HIPAA. You can freely refer to Dr. Jonathon Doe or Nurse Jane Smith in your notes. In fact, doing so can eliminate some of the confusion that comes inherently with trying to decipher the contents of a patient's chart if an auditor digs through your notes years in the future.

Streamline the Documentation Process

Chapter Overview

- **Keep notes as events unfold.**
- **Chart in real-time as much as possible.**
- **Copy and paste from templates to save keystrokes.**

Keep Notes

Having a pen and paper handy to jot times, dosages, witnesses, and patient statements down for later usually pays off. In the absence of a pen and paper, write data on your gloves, paper towels, or alcohol swab wrappers, then do your best to transcribe the data from those makeshift notepads as soon as possible before they are misplaced.

Chart Early and Often

It can be more than easy to get swept up in the chaos of a shift, only to realize three hours later that you're far behind on charting everything that has been happening. If you have access to mobile workstations on wheels, chart at the bedside whenever possible. Even if you just have a minute here or there while your patient is using the restroom or taking a handful of pills one by one, those minutes add up and help tackle the never-ending list of data points you need to document.

Specific to narrative notes, being able to type quickly without looking at the keyboard is a huge timesaver. If you're a nurse who has to type two fingers at a time with a great deal of concentration, writing the necessary narrative notes will simply take longer. Learning efficient typing habits can help save immense amounts of time on your shift.

Create a Template

I want to preface this section with a disclaimer: I have heard the argument from nurse managers that copying a pasting from a template is like asking to make an error in a chart. I understand it can seem easy to copy and paste a paragraph into a note, and then forget to modify it to fit your specific patient.

My rebuttal to this argument is that nursing requires attention to detail for all important aspects of the job, and nurses are trusted to carry out those tasks even though they require focus. Pills are routinely stocked in a dosage other than whatever is ordered for your patient, requiring you to cut it in half to give the patient the right dose. Medications are available in liquid form, requiring careful measurement. Pediatric doses are calculated based on weight, requiring a whole math equation to ensure that the littlest patients receive the right dose. I think nurses can handle pasting a few lines into a chart and modifying them as necessary.

For my templates, I like having a Word document available on my computer that can be easily edited as I think of time-saving sentences to add, or reorganized if I find myself scrolling to find one specific paragraph multiple times a shift. If you are not able to keep a Word document saved to your workstation, consider using the draft of an email that you can pull up whenever you need it.

Use the examples I've provided later in this book to help you build your own templates. A template can be as much or as little as you find helpful. Ensure that it is easy for you to identify the areas that need to be edited to describe the individual patient on whom you are charting.

For example, your assumption of care note may begin, "Received report from John Doe, RN."

A template for that sentence could be written one of several ways:

1. Received report from **XXXX**, RN.
2. Received report from
3. Received report from **NURSE'S NAME.**
4. Received report from **(nurse)** in **(department).**

Create your templates in ways that you find the most helpful.

Prefer a ready-to-use version available as an instant download? I made my 15-page working template available to you at **www.zephryco.com** as part of a bundle of tools that will save you time and headaches right away.

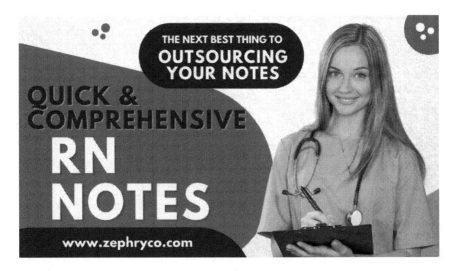

Abbreviations

Chapter Overview:

- **Use only approved abbreviations at your facility.**
- **When in doubt, spell it out.**
- **Never use abbreviations on the "do not use" list.**

The Joint Commission determines acceptable abbreviations. Understanding when to use abbreviations is best summarized in six words: **When in doubt, spell it out.**

There is a list of approved abbreviations, and it changes over time. Find out if your facility has a current list of approved abbreviations.

You will see many abbreviations used in my examples. There is no guarantee that the abbreviations in the following examples are on the current list of approved abbreviations. As you read some of my example, decide for yourself whether the information being relayed is clear, or if you would find it easier to decipher what happened if the abbreviations had been spelled out.

The Joint Commission states that an individual facility may have their own standardized abbreviations for use within the facility, which should be easily accessed by all staff. While the running list of abbreviations you may use could change or differ, there is a set list of abbreviations that should never be used.

If your facility does not have a prominently displayed or easily accessible list of approved abbreviations, ask your chain of management for one.

The "<u>do not use</u>" list includes:

- Do not use U or u in place of **unit**

- Do not use IU in place of **International Unit**

- Do not use Q.D., QD, q.d., or qd in place of **daily**

- Do not use Q.O.D., QOD, q.o.d, or qod in place of **every other day**

- Do not use a trailing zero **(X.0 mg)**

- *Alternatively, you must use a leading zero for decimal points* **(0.X mg)**

- Do not use MS, MSO4 or MgSO4 in place of **morphine sulfate** or **magnesium sulfate**

Daily Notes

Chapter Overview:

- **Include assumption of care and handoff notes daily for each patient.**
- **Summarize interactions with providers.**
- **Write additional notes for any information not otherwise captured in flowsheets.**

Is there a set checklist of notes you should complete every shift for every patient? The short answer is that it varies. Having worked both day shift and night shift on med/surg, ortho, pediatrics, infusion therapy, and rehab, the only constant that I can state from my multiple prior positions is that there were no two shifts that were the same. It was difficult to predict how my day would go, what patients would be admitted, and what might go wrong (usually, a lot). Narrative notes are free-texted for a reason: they need to be tailored to a specific patient in a specific situation. While I do utilize the templates that I previously mentioned to prevent redundant typing and create a basic structure to build my notes around, rarely have I saved and submitted two notes that are identical. However, there are patterns that present themselves and repeat regularly.

ASSUMPTION OF CARE

For example, I try to enter an *assumption of care* note for every patient that I receive a report about. After the off-going nurse gives me a report, I copy and paste my template for my *assumption of care* note into a narrative section of the chart and then modify the words and phrases necessary to make the note 100 percent accurate for the individual patient.

If the patient's chart is designed to tell a story about the patient's status and plan of care on any given shift, the *assumption of care* note is like the introduction. I can summarize the *assumption of care* note in a few words: "Here's a snapshot of the patient exactly as they were when I started my shift."

Assumption of Care Note Example

Received report from Lena Empyema, RN. Patient resting in bed with eyes closed, regular chest rise and fall, no sign of acute distress. Last set of VS taken at 0600 stable, WNL. See VS flowsheet. IVF infusing at prescribed rate, IV site without redness, edema, or streaking, dressing CDI. Nasal cannula remains in place, current oxygen flow at 2 lpm via NC, SpO2 > 90%. Bed is in lowest, locked position with side rails up x2. Patient belongings at bedside. Call light in reach.

HANDOFF REPORT

Similarly, a handoff report is like the conclusion paragraph of an essay that ties up any loose ends. Writing a quick handoff narrative note after giving report to the oncoming nurse provides a snapshot of the patient's status as you left them in the capable hands of the next shift.

End of Shift Hand-off Note Example

Gave report to Lena Empyema, RN. Patient resting in chair at bedside. Regular chest rise and fall, no sign of acute distress. All patient's questions answered prior to shift change. Vital signs stable, WNL. See vitals flow sheet. IVF infusing at prescribed rate. IV site WNL, no redness, no edema, dressing CDI. Current oxygen flow at 2 lpm via NC and SpO2 > 90%. Non-slip socks on bilateral feet. Call light within reach. Patient has been using call light appropriately throughout shift. Bed is in lowest, locked position for patient return. Patient belongings in reach.

PROVIDER AT BEDSIDE/COMMUNICATION WITH PROVIDER

You may not communicate with a provider on every shift about every patient, but I'm including this example under the context of a note that you should write every shift because you likely will talk to a provider at some point during your shift about one or more of your patients.

Writing a note after an interaction with a provider helps ensure adequate communication. When the provider is at a patient's bedside, it is good practice to listen to what the provider is telling the patient whenever possible. Doing so can help you stay up to date on a patient's plan of care, and give you an opportunity to ensure that all of the patient's questions are answered.

After the provider talks to the patient, a quick note summarizing the conversation helps ensure the chart is up-to-date in real time even if the provider isn't able to enter new orders for a few hours, as an example.

Alternatively, speaking to a provider on the phone also warrants a quick note. Again, a simple summary of the conversation can help not only other team members stay aware of the patient's plan of care, but could serve as a reminder to a provider if new orders or follow-ups are necessary. Hospital providers are constantly pulled in just as many directions as nurses, and it can take time for a provider to sit down at a computer and catch up on his or her own documentation. A quick note summarizing a conversation that happened earlier in the day can be helpful for both parties.

Provider at Bedside Note Example

Dr. Gudhelth rounding on patient at bedside. Provided an update to patient regarding plan of care, including an update about most recent lab and imaging results. Performed assessment. Answered all patient's questions regarding plan of care. Patient's spouse at bedside. Dr. Gudhelth also answered all spouse's questions. Modified medication orders per patient request, see ORDERS in patient chart.

EXAMPLES FOR COMMON OCCURRENCES ON AN INPATIENT WARD

DISCLAIMER: *The sample entries in the following pages are* **examples**. *While I drew on professional experience to write them, any descriptions of patients have either been fabricated or are the composite of multiple experiences rolled into one.*

Every nurse documents a little differently. Explaining situations and occurrences differently does not mean you are wrong, or vice versa. Further, each patient is an individual and requires some personalized touches. Every situation is different, and rarely does a medical scenario unfold in a textbook fashion. These example are designed to provide the structure for narrative notes, but narrative notes that you write about your patients will likely not be exactly the same.

New Admission

Chapter Overview:

- **Write one note about the report received on an incoming patient.**
- **Write an additional note for the assumption of care when the patient physically arrives.**
- **Inventory belongings without assigning perceived values to items.**

New admissions throughout your shift usually require a couple of narrative notes to capture the entire beginning of their story.

I have found it easiest to write a minimum of two notes for a new admission. When I receive report from another department or facility who is sending the patient to me, I write a note detailing the information from that report. This is separate from the assumption of care note, which I write when the patient physically arrives on the unit and I begin caring for him or her.

The assumption of care note for a new admission generally looks different from an assumption of care note that I write when I take over a patient from a previous shift. Admitting a new patient requires more education for the patient and his or her family, sometimes requires a new IV to be initiated, and requires inventorying belongings that the patient brings to the hospital.

Some hospitals have their own intake form for an inventory of belongings. If your specific place of employment requires a different format, your assumption of care notes for new admissions may look different. The part that shouldn't look different, however, is the phrasing. Many nurses mistakenly mis-inventory items, such as gold watches or diamond rings. It's not within your scope to be able to identify precious metals or expensive items, so an inventory of items should be very simplistic, such as a "yellow metal watch" and a "metal ring with a clear stone."

NEW ADMISSION
From Emergency Department

Example of Report

Received report from Run Kodez, RN, in ED. Patient arrived to ED this morning at 0900 complaining of RLQ abdominal pain x3 days. Patient accompanied by spouse. Patient reports onset of nausea/vomiting around 0300 today accompanied by intensifying of RLQ pain. Patient reports he took OTC ibuprofen at home, estimates dose at 800mg, with no relief. Since admission to ED, patient has received 4 mg morphine via IV and 4 mg ondansetron via IV. Pain decreased from 8/10 to 4/10 per patient report and is tolerable. Nausea/vomiting well controlled at this time. Patient s/p CT of abdomen, results indicating acute appendicitis per radiology report. Patient being admitted to ward with 18g IV to R AC, received 1 L NS in ED, spouse remains at bedside. Plan to proceed to surgery for appendectomy at 0500. Will await patient arrival.

Example of Assumption of Care

Patient arrival to Med/Surg ward at 2311 via wheelchair accompanied by ED staff. Spouse at patient's side. Patient able to transfer self to bed with no assistance required. Patient states he last voided at 2300, no urge to void at this time. IV assessment WNL, dressing CDI. All patient's questions answered upon arrival to ward. No acute distress. Initiated all orders, see ORDERS in patient chart.

NEW ADMISSION
From Post-Anesthesia Care Unit

Example of Report

Received report from Surg McGee in PACU. Patient s/p appendectomy and recovering in PACU. In OR, per nurse McGee, patient received 1 L LR, 25 mcg Fentanyl at 0854, 4 mg Zofran at 0855, and 1 g Ancef at 0859. Patient has 4 laparoscopic incisions to abdomen, Dermabond applied to all, all approximated and OTA. Patient vomited 200 mL upon arrival to PACU at 0910. In PACU, patient received 25 mg Phenergan at 0915. No emesis since administration of Phenergan. Patient has received a total of 2 mg Dilaudid via IV in PACU, last dose at 0930. Patient reports pain at 2/10 and tolerable. Tolerated sips of water. Oxygen above 90% on room air. See VITALS in patient chart for all vitals taken in PACU, last set stable and WNL. Friend of patient at bedside will accompany patient to ward. Will await patient arrival.

Example of Assumption of Care

Patient arrival to ward at 1005 on gurney accompanied by PACU staff. Patient in no acute distress at time of arrival, pain tolerable. Patient able to transfer self to bed with minimal assistance. Arrived with patent 18 g IV in left hand, site findings WNL, dressing CDI. Initiated IVF at prescribed rate. VS taken immediately upon arrival, see VS in EMR. Patient reports pain as 3/10 and tolerable. Patient with urge to void. Urinal provided, 300 mL yellow urine voided, DTV met.

NEW ADMISSION
From Clinic

Example of Report

Report received from Tellie Helth, RN. Patient arrived to clinic appointment this morning at 1015 to address increasing SOA. In clinic, patient diagnosed with asthma exacerbation. An albuterol treatment and a Duoneb treatment both given to patient in clinic. Patient declines improvement in feeling SOA, Nurse Helth reports initial SpO2 87% on room air. Patient responsive to 1 L oxygen via NC, patient to 93% with supplemental oxygen. Per Nurse Helth, patient with expiratory wheezes in all lung fields and decreased lung sounds in RLL and LLL. Patient denies pain. Past medical history includes asthma and allergies to dust, peanuts, penicillins, and lisinopril. Patient unable to identify exacerbating factors. Will await patient arrival.

Example of Assumption of care

Patient arrival to ward at 1445 in wheelchair accompanied by clinic staff. Patient on 1 lpm via NC, SpO2 above 90%. VS stable and WNL, see VS in patient chart. Patient transferred self to bed. Denies pain and unmet needs. Patient arrived without IV access. Patient belonging and call bell within reach, bed in lowest, locked position, no acute distress.

Example of Order Clarification

Paged physician to clarify orders. Patient has IV Solumedrol ordered but does not have IV access and does not have an order to obtain IV access. Further, patient states that he takes Claritin qAM, but does not have Claritin ordered. Dr.

Gudhelth returned paged at 1510. New order for qAM Claritin, see MAR. Further, Dr. Gudhelth confirmed order for IV Solumedrol, entered new order to initiate PIV access.

Inventory of Belongings Note Example

Patient arrived to unit with one tan fabric tote bag in her possession. Patient unpacked tote bag for inventorying purposes. Inside tote, patient possesses a purple pillowcase, a black comb, a pair of socks, an iPhone charger (white, 6 feet long), and a yellow metal watch with an elastic band. All items left in possession of patient. Provided falls risk education regarding socks and provided patient with a new pair of nonslip socks. Patient verbalized understanding to wear nonslip socks when out of bed.

GENERAL SURGICAL
DIAGNOSIS EXAMPLES

By LENA EMPYEMA | www.zephryco.com

General Pre-Op Example

Patient has been NPO since midnight. Last meal at 1930 yesterday, last sip of water at 2330 yesterday. Patient received one dose of IV morphine at 0330, see MAR. Chlorhexadine bath given at 0500. Bedside report given to OR nurse Beta Dine, RN. Patient transported to OR accompanied by OR staff for surgeon to obtain informed consents.

General Post-Op Example

Received report from Wake Andsip, RN in PACU. Patient s/p cholecystectomy. Per Andsip, RN, patient received 1g Ancef prior to procedure in OR. Total of 1 L LR infused in OR. 500 mL LR infused in PACU. Patient received a total of 50 mcg Fentanyl and 4 mg Zofran in PACU, now rating pain 3/10 and tolerable. Last dose of Fentanyl at 1115, see MAR. Patient tolerating ice chips without nausea or emesis. No urine output since surgery, patient will be due to void 6 hours post-op per orders at 1600. 5 lap sites to abdomen, all closed with Dermabond and open to air, approximated, and without drainage, per PACU nurse. Patient transported to ward on gurney accompanied by PACU staff. Patient transferred self to ward bed. No acute distress. Pain now 5/10, still tolerable at this time, patient states he does not want pain medication at this time. Initiated IVF at prescribed rate. Ensured SCDs are on bilateral lower extremities and functioning properly. Patient denies unmet needs at this time. Bed in lowest locked position, side rails up x2, call light in reach.

S/p Bariatric Surgery Post-op Report Example

Patient is a 37 y/o female s/p lap sleeve procedure. BMI 41. Patient with 10-year history of obesity complicated by Type II DM (non-insulin-dependent), hypertension, hyperlipidemia, hypercholesterolemia, GERD, Irritable Bowel Syndrome, depression, anxiety, and panic disorder. Lap sites x3, closed with Dermabond, OTA, approximated, no drainage, no odor, no edema, no erythema. JP drain to RUQ, gauze CDI, bulb secured to gown and draining small amount of serosanguinous drainage.

S/p Gynecological Surgery Example

Received report from Requuver Master, RN, in PACU. Patient is a 41 y/o female s/p vaginal hysterectomy with no visible external incision sites. History of G2P2, both vaginal deliveries. Heavy vaginal bleeding has been baseline for 6 months. Scant sanguinous spotting on pad in PACU. Patient received 25 mcg Fentanyl at 1455, 4 mg Zofran at 1510, 2 mg Morphine at 1540, pain now tolerable at 3/10, no nausea/vomiting. No external drains.

TRANSFERS & TRANSPORTS
EXAMPLES

Overview of Narrative Notes About Transfers:

- When applicable, document use of gait belt, walker, cane, or other assistive devices
- Document extent of assistance patient needs to safely ambulate.
- Include reference to PT/OT consults as applicable.
- Minimize trip hazards in patient room and document your efforts to keep the path to the exits and bathroom clear.

Overview of Narrative Notes About Transports:

- For patients dependent on supplemental oxygen, ensure that portable tanks are used and document their use and flow.
- For high risk or unstable patients, an RN should stay with the patient when off the unit, and the note should include mention of the RN staying with the patient.
- Document the assistive device used to transport patient if applicable, such as a wheelchair.
- Include in the note the summary of the patient's safe return to the room.
- If there are deviations or adverse events, document what happened, the actions taken, and the outcome.

Example of Ambulation

Educated patient about safe ambulation with two staff members assisting. Patient verbalized understanding of use of gait belt, nonslip socks, and walker. RN and CNA at patient bedside to assist patient. Patient able to sit at edge of bed and dangle legs with moderate assistance. Gait belt secured around patient's waist, non-slip socks to bilateral feet. Walker placed at bedside and adjusted to appropriate height for patient. Patient denies dizziness and light-headedness while sitting at edge of bed. Patient assisted to stand with moderate assistance from staff. Patient demonstrated safe use of walker. With staff maintaining grip on gait belt, patient ambulated approximately ten yards, then returned to bed without adverse event. Gait belt removed. Patient reported increased pain to lower back after returning to bed. See MAR for PRN medications administered. No acute distress, call button placed within patient reach, patient belongings within reach at bedside.

Example of Transporting Patient Off Ward for Imaging

Per physician's orders, patient to undergo CXR / MRI / CT. Phone call placed to imaging unit, team is ready to receive patient for imaging study at this time. RN explained plan of care to patient, answered all of patient's questions, patient verbalized understanding of POC. Portable oxygen tank at back of wheelchair, patient will remain on 2 lpm via NC for transport and during procedure. CNA and RN at bedside to assist with transfer to wheelchair. Gait belt placed around patient's waist and non-slip socks placed on bilateral feet. Patient able to stand and pivot to chair with minimal assist. No acute distress. Patient transported to imaging in wheelchair accompanied by ward staff.

INITIATING INVASIVE DEVICES

Example of IV Initiation

Updated patient on plan of care, to include initiating IV access and initiating IV Solumedrol for asthma exacerbation. Patient verbalized understanding of plan. RN explained procedure for inserting IV. All of patient's questions answered prior to IV insertion. All supplies gathered at bedside. Confirmed that patient has no limb restrictions. Identified vein for IV insertion. Applied tourniquet. Inserted 20 g IV into left anterior forearm. Blood return verified, 10 mL saline flush per protocol. IV flushed without resistance. Secured IV with plastic tape and IV dressing. Dated IV dressing. Initiated IVF at KVO rate of 20 mL LR/hour. Patient tolerated procedure well without adverse event. Will administer IV Solumedrol after pharmacy verifies medication order and supplies IVPB. Patient has no further questions at this time.

Example of Venipuncture

Explained need to collect CBC and CMP. Patient verbalized understanding. Gathered necessary equipment at the bedside. Explained procedure to patient, answered all of patient's questions, patient verbalized understanding of plan of care. Paused administration of IV fluids and selected venipuncture site on arm opposite where IV fluids have been infusing. Prepared puncture site with alcohol and allowed skin to dry. Applied tourniquet, inserted 20g IV catheter using proper technique without resistance, obtained blood sample on first attempt. Filled gold top tube then lavender top tube. Removed tourniquet. Applied clean gauze dressing, secured with self-adherent wrap. Patient tolerated procedure without adverse event. Labelled tubes at bedside with patient name and DOB. Placed tubes in biohazard bag and transported to lab immediately.

Example of Foley Placement

Reviewed order to place indwelling Foley catheter. Gathered necessary equipment at the bedside and explained procedure to patient. Answered all patient's questions. Patient verbalized understanding of plan of care. CNA Lisa at bedside to assist with patient positioning. Patient assisted into supine position. Labium cleansed thoroughly using a single downward stroke with povidone iodine swabs per aseptic protocol. 18 Fr single lumen Foley catheter inserted into urethra on first attempt using aseptic technique with positive return of clear yellow urine. Balloon inflated with 10 mLs normal saline. Secured Foley to left thigh with adhesive Statlock device. Placed urine drainage bag below level of bladder on bed frame hook off of floor. Assisted patient into comfortable position. Educated patient to use call light for assistance and to not get out of bed alone due to new trip hazard. Patient verbalized understanding.

Example of NG Insertion

Physician at bedside verbalizing order for new NG tube placement. Gathered necessary equipment at the bedside. John Smith, RN, assisted patient into High Fowler's position. Measured length of NG tube using nose to earlobe to xyphoid process and cut to length. Using proper technique, inserted 16 Fr single lumen levin tube through left nare to posterior nasopharynx. Patient able to swallow sips of water. Used irrigation syringe to push air into tube, auscultated bubbles in upper left quadrant of abdomen. Secured tube to bridge of nose with silk tape. Per physician at bedside, x-ray to be obtained prior to NG tube use.

ORTHOPEDIC DIAGNOSES

S/p Total Knee Arthroplasty

Patient s/p TKA to right knee. Patient with history of LTKA and is familiar with procedures. Dressing to knee CDI. Ice applied to dorsal surface of knee. RLE warm with full sensation per patient report. Patient able to wiggle all toes. Dorsalis pedis pulses +3 and equal bilaterally. RLE warm to touch, color of skin normal for race. No pillow under operative knee. Walker and gait belt at bedside. All patient's questions answered at this time.

S/p Total Hip Arthroplasty

Patient s/p total hip arthroplasty to left hip. Patient with history of DMII, HTN, HLD, OSA, and OA. Last A1C 5.9, last serum blood glucose 110, patient well-controlled with diet and PO Metformin at home. Patient arrival to ward with abductor pillow in place, toes pointed straight up, nothing under operative leg. Walker and gait belt at bedside. Patient reminded to not bend at the hips more than 90 degrees. Patient verbalized understanding of education and precautions. Provided patient with incentive spirometer and educated on its use. Patient able to demonstrate use of IS and verbalize understanding of using it 10 times per hour.

S/p Total Shoulder Arthroplasty

Patient arrival to ward s/p total shoulder arthroplasty to right shoulder. Sling in place and adjusted to proper fit. Non-weight bearing status of right shoulder confirmed with patient upon arrival to ward, patient verbalized understanding to not use right limb. Limb restriction sign placed on door and over bed, limb restriction band placed on right wrist. 20 g IV in L AC, initiated fluids at prescribed rate. Patient with pain 7/10, not tolerable at this time. Non-pharmacological interventions failed to improve pain management. PRN oxycodone administered to patient, see MAR. 60 minutes after administration, patient reports pain as a tolerable 5/10. PT at bedside to initiate therapy with patient. Patient ambulated to bathroom with gait belt secured around waist, voided 500 mL amber urine, met DTV s/p surgical procedure.

Examples of Other Orthopedic Assessments

Circulation in surgical extremity example

Pulses strong and equal bilaterally. Patient able to wiggle all toes/fingers. Full and equal sensation to limbs bilaterally. Limbs warm to palpation. Capillary refill less than 3 seconds. No mottling. Dorsiflexion and plantar flexion intact bilaterally. Patient denies chest pain, SOA. Pain 4/10 and tolerable at this time.

Example of patient working with physical therapy

Physical therapy with patient for duration of 1 hour. Per PTA report, patient able to ambulate 10 yards using walker and gait belt with minimal assistance. No adverse events during PT session. Pain elevated to 5/10 after PT session and PRN Motrin administered, see MAR. Patient returned to bed after PT session, ice to operative limb, assessment findings WNL.

Example of patient working with occupational therapy

Occupational therapy at bedside to assess and treat patient. IV disconnected from IVF. Protective plastic cover applied to IV and secured with water resistant tape. Protective plastic covering also applied to incision site and secured with water resistant tape. Patient showered with assistance of OT. Per OT report, patient required moderate assistance to stand and wash lower extremities bilaterally. No adverse events. Patient returned safely to bed. IVF reinitiated at prescribed rate.

MEDICAL DIAGNOSES

Gynecological Diagnosis

Status Update for Patient with Heavy Vaginal Bleeding

Patient has saturated 2 pads in 6 hours. Parameters state to notify provider when 1 pad is saturated per hour for 2 hours in a row. Provider not notified at this time. VSS. Patient denies light-headedness, chest pain, dizziness, and SOA. Provided patient with more pads and disposable mesh underwear.

Urological Diagnoses

Status Update for a Patient with Recurring UTIs

Assisted patient to restroom. Educated patient to wipe front to back when performing perineal hygiene. Urine in toilet clear yellow. Patient denies dysuria. Green exudate present in patient's underwear. Provided patient with disposable mesh underwear. Notified provider via telephone of discharge. No new orders at this time.

Rhabdomyolysis Note Example

Patient admitted to ward for 6 hours before voiding into urinal. Urine dark brown in color, unable to assess clarity due to color. Amount totalled 90 mL. Average urine output currently 15 mL/hour. Provider aware that patient is not voiding an average of 30 mL/hour. If urinary production has not increased by 1800, provider requested phone call.

Gastrointestinal Diagnosis

Status Update on Patient with Suspected Small Bowel Obstruction

Patient reports persistent pain in right lower quadrant. Bowel sounds equally hypoactive in all quadrants. Patient denies passing flatus. Cannot recall last time flatus was passed. Last bowel movement at least four days ago. Bowel movement at that time was small and hard per patient report. Patient reports a history of a small bowel obstruction approximately ten years ago, cannot recall what treatment she received, cannot recall how long she was hospitalized. Record not available. Patient with NPO orders but was sipping water from sink. Educated patient about NPO orders. Notified physician of assessment findings, patient reported history, and noncompliance with diet orders. New order for abdominal x-ray.

Patients at High Risk for Falls

Nearly every patient is at risk for falls to some degree, but some are certainly at higher risk than others.

Where applicable, include short blurbs about nursing interventions taken to minimize falls risks.

- For insulin-dependent diabetic patients, document any snacks or food given to the patient at the same time as sliding scale insulin coverage.
- For all falls risks patients, document that the call bell is within reach and that the patient was reminded to use it before getting out of bed, the gait belt is at the bedside, the placement of the walker or assistive devices, and the bed in the lowest locked position.

ADVERSE EVENTS

Example of IV Infiltration

Patient used call bell to notify nursing staff of pain at IV site. IV site edematous with slight erythema, firm to palpation. IVF immediately stopped. Removed PIV and applied pressure for 60 seconds before placing pressure dressing using clean gauze and a self-adherent wrap. Educated patient to leave dressing in place for at least 30 minutes. Patient verbalized understanding. Obtained ice pack to apply to site. Educated patient to apply ice pack to edematous site for 15 minutes then provide 15 minutes of rest from cold therapy, during which time skin should remain OTA. Patient verbalized understanding of instructions. Confirmed that no vesicants were infusing at time of suspected infiltration, only LR as prescribed IVF was running. Obtained supplies at bedside to initiate new PIV. Applied tourniquet to arm opposite the site where IV suspected to have infiltrated. First attempt failed to secure IV access, second attempt successful at establishing IV access in R hand using 20 g catheter. Confirmed blood return and saline flush without resistance. Secured IV with tape and dressing. Patient tolerated procedure well, no adverse event. Tourniquet removed promptly after securing IV access.

Example of a Potential Allergic Reaction

During routine hourly rounding, patient reported intense pruritus. Blotchy red pattern observed on skin proximal to IV site where Levaquin was infusing. Immediately stopped IV infusion of antibiotic. Confirmed allergy status with patient. Patient stated she has no known medication allergies. Obtained set of VS. All VS WNL, see VS in EMR. Immediately notified provider of pruritic rash on the extremity where medication was infusing. Telephone order transcribed from Dr. Gudhelth to administer 50 mg IV diphenhydramine and discontinue further administration of Levaquin. RN accessed Pyxis, found no diphenhydramine available for patient. Called pharmacy and relayed telephone order for medication due to potential reaction to Levaquin. Per Sylvia in pharmacy, RN okay to override diphenhydramine in Pyxis to facilitate rapid administration. Overrode medication, then confirmed correct medication with Norma Vitalis, RN. 50 mg diphenhydramine diluted in 10 mL NS, then pushed over 2 minutes into patient's patent IV with patient consent. Patient tolerated administration well and experienced relief of pruritus. No additional adverse symptoms reported, patient denies SOA, denies chest pain, denies lightheadedness, denies dizziness, and denies gastrointestinal upset.

Examples of a Potential Reaction to Blood Product Administration

At approximately 1315, within the first ten minutes of initiating blood administration, patient experienced increase in basal temperature from 97.9 degrees F to 100.2 degrees F, more than 2 degrees. Per protocol, blood products immediately stopped from infusing. NS initiated through IV at a rate of 100 mL/hour per protocol. RN immediately collected 8 mL blood into lavender top tube and assisted patient to restroom to collect urine sample. Both blood and urine sample placed in biohazard bags and labelled with two patient identifiers at bedside. Disconnected all blood tubing from IV pump and placed remaining blood products and IV lines in biohazard bag. Gave blood product, lines, blood sample, and urine sample to CNA for immediate transport to lab. Paged provider. Dr. Gudhelth returned page at 1330. RN communicated findings and actions taken to Dr. Gudhelth. New orders at this time to administer 25 mg IV Benadryl to patient. Order placed in EMR, medication drawn from Pyxis per orders and administered to patient diluted in 10 mL NS slow push to patient. Patient continues to report experiencing no other adverse symptoms.

Examples of Falls

Fall without Obvious Injury

Around 1400, patient requested to ambulate to bathroom. Patient has been a minimal, one-person assist for transfers for the duration of her four-day hospital stay. RN placed gait belt around patient's waist securely and ensured that non-skid socks were well-fitted to each foot. Patient began ambulating to bathroom without the assistance of walker or cane per baseline. When patient approached the threshold at the door of the bathroom, patient tripped and fell forward. RN's hand remained on gait belt, but RN was unable to stop the fall. Patient landed on her knees. RN called for assistance. Two additional staff members, Claire Jones, CNA, and Wendy Johnson, CNA, arrived in the patient's room with a wheelchair. Patient assisted to her feet. VS taken immediately, VS WNL and at baseline for patient, see VS in EMR. Provider notified. Provider stated since the fall was witnessed and patient did not hit her head, no orders for CT or other imaging. Provider stated he will come see patient to assess any injury to her lower extremities. After the fall, patient assisted safely to bedside commode to void, and returned to bed safely. PRN Tylenol provided for aching left knee following the fall, see MAR.

Fall with Possible Injury

Patient with history of quadriplegia requires total assistance with the aid of at least two staff members at baseline. Staff have been using a Hoyer lift for duration of patient admission to move patient from bed to power chair. Around 0815, accompanied CNA Claire Jones into patient room to assist patient into chair for therapy. Sling placed adequately underneath patient and Hoyer lift used to move patient from bed. Patient positioned over chair and staff lowered patient into chair. Sling was unhooked from Hoyer lift. After sling was unhooked, patient slid further forward in the chair and fell onto the floor. Witnessed patient strike head on the foot rest of the power chair. Small amount of bleeding present to laceration on scalp. Additional staff called for assistance and two RNs, Jacob Jacobsen, RN, and John Jonathon, RN, entered room to help. VS taken while patient remained on floor, pillow placed under his head for comfort, and pressure applied to laceration using clean gauze. Patient's heart rate to 120 bpm from baseline in 90s (see vitals flow sheet) and blood pressure decreased from to 88/47 from baseline (see vitals flow sheet) . Charge nurse immediately called provider to update on events. Dr. Nyce arrived at patient bedside as nursing staff was repositioning Hoyer sling to lift patient into bed. Verbal orders at bedside to obtain CT of head which Dr. Nyce later entered into EMR. Patient transported to imaging on bed accompanied by two RNs. Uneventful transfer from bed to CT machine.

Follow Up for Fall with Possible Injury

Patient returned to ward on bed. Per Dr. Nyce, CT results showed new subdural hematoma. Patient's VS without improvement from earlier set taken immediately after fall. BP remains in the high 80s/40s (see vitals flow sheet for specific values), heart rate remains in the 120s (see VS in flow sheet). Verbal order from Dr. Nyce to initiate IVF bolus of NS, 1 L to be infused rapidly over 30 minutes. Initiated fluid bolus. Verbal order to transfer patient to higher level of care. Report called to ICU nurse Leva Fedd, RN. Patient transported to ICU on bed accompanied by two ward staff. Patient arrived to ICU responsive and oriented x4, VS remained at new baseline since fall (see VS in EMR) and Leva Fedd, RN assumed care of patient.

Example of Leaving Against Medical Advice

Around 2030, patient approached nurse's station and stated, "I'm leaving. I'm done waiting for the doctor. I just thought you should know." RN asked patient if something was wrong. Patient stated, "I've been here three days, I've seen the doctor twice, they don't know what's wrong, and I'm going to another hospital." RN explained that test results were still pending, and that the provider would use lab results to help determine patient's diagnosis. Patient began yelling, "I don't care, I'm leaving!" All of his belongings were packed and in a bag on his shoulder. Patient walked towards the exit. Followed patient, asking him to please wait just a moment while charge nurse paged provider about patient's concerns. Patient refused, walking towards the elevators. RN explained that patient had the right to leave the hospital and was not being held against his will, but that a signature AMA paperwork would be necessary. Patient agreed. RN provided paperwork to patient while charge nurse paged provider. Provider arrived on ward rapidly to speak to patient. Patient continued to insist that he was leaving the hospital. Provider explained that patient would be leaving against medical advice, carrying with it the risk of serious injury up to and including death. Patient verbalized understanding and signed AMA paperwork. PIV removed, dressed with gauze and self-adherent wrap. Educated patient to leave pressure dressing in place for at least thirty minutes. Patient verbalized understanding of teaching. Patient left the hospital with all of his belongings.

Examples of Noncompliance with Provider's Orders

Diet/Fluid Restriction

Patient with history of congestive heart failure, currently admitted for CHF exacerbation, and restricted to 1500 mg sodium per day as part of treatment protocol. Educated patient on sodium restriction and explained where to find sodium content information on inpatient menu. Discussed where to find sodium content on nutrition labels in grocery stores and healthy food options low in sodium. Patient has been ordering foods low in sodium from inpatient menu. In addition to hospital meals, patient's spouse has been visiting patient twice per day with bags of fast food. Empty fast food containers found in trash twice this shift. Patient denies eating the food in the bags. Assessment reveals pitting edema in bilateral lower extremities. Edema was 2+ this morning, now is 3+, see assessment flow sheet for details. Patient exhibiting increased shortness of breath and crackles in lower lung fields bilaterally. Notified provider of changes in assessment findings. Patient continuing to receive furosemide as ordered. Reminded patient of the risks associated with consuming excessive amounts of sodium. Patient verbalized understanding.

Medication Refusal

Patient ordered to receive metoprolol and HCTZ this morning at 0800. Nursing staff entered room shortly after 0800 to administer medication. Patient refused, stating, "I do not want to take any more pills." Last BP elevated above baseline, see vitals flow sheet for values. RN educated patient on the purpose of metoprolol and HCTZ and informed patient that his BP is elevated. Educated patient on the risks of uncontrolled high blood pressure. Patient again stated, "I am not taking any more pills." RN left patient room to treat other patients, then returned at 0845 to offer medications once again. Again, patient refused. Paged provider at 0850. Dr. Gudhelth returned page at 0905 and RN updated provider on patient refusal and VS. No new orders. Dr. Gudhelth stated he will come talk to patient later in the morning.

Examples of Arrhythmias on Telemetry Monitor

Actual new onset, asymptomatic

Telemetry technician called primary care nurse at 1100 stating that patient's monitor showed trigeminy. Immediately entered patient room to assess patient. Patient denied chest pain, denied chest pressure, denied shortness of breath, denied dizziness, and denied light-headedness. Patient denies any abnormal symptoms aside from LLQ abdominal pain which patient has been experiencing intermittently since admission (provider aware per last progress note). Vital signs obtained, all VS at baseline for patient. All previous EKGs showed normal sinus rhythm. Paged provider at 1115, provider returned page at 1118, RN informed provider of new onset trigeminy. No new orders at this time.

Actual new onset arrhythmia, symptomatic

Telemetry technician notified RN around 1400 that telemetry strip showed supraventricular tachycardia. Immediately entered patient room to assess and found patient reclined in bedside chair, diaphoretic, and pale. Patient's respiratory rate was increased from a baseline of 16 to a rate of 22 (see vitals flow sheet). Immediately initiated Rapid Response team for acute changes in patient status. RRT arrived to bedside at 1407. RN gave summarized report of patient history and onset of SVT to ICU RN, Letz Savem. RRT assumed care of patient, initiated order set per protocol, and transported patient to higher level of care. Patient transported off of ward to ICU at 1420.

Apparent new onset of arrhythmia, result of equipment malfunction

Telemetry technician called RN at 1300 to report ventricular tachycardia on monitor. Immediately entered patient room to assess. Patient resting comfortably in bed, no sign of acute distress, regular chest rise and fall. RN awoke patient to assess for chest pain. Patient denied chest pain and denied pressure, denied shortness of air. RN assessed telemetry leads. RLL disconnected from electrode. RN replaced electrode. Telemetry monitor now shows NSR with a rate of 70.

Example of Administration of Naloxone for Overdose

Patient's orders for up to 10 mg oxycodone available q4 hours and up to 0.6 mg hydromorphone available q2 hours. Patient has been requesting all available pain medications regularly for uncontrolled 10/10 pain, see MAR and VS flow sheet. Around 0200, entered room to find patient supine in bed and difficult to arouse. At this time, respiratory rate was 10 breaths per minute. RN sternal rubbed patient, patient responded with moan, but patient did not open eyes and did not speak any discernible words. Full set of VS obtained at 0203. See vitals flow sheet for values. Patient placed on 2 lpm of oxygen therapy, bringing SpO2 above 90%. Patient had no oxygen requirement previously. Standing order from Dr. Gudhelth to administer 1 mg naloxone for a patient prescribed opioids with a respiratory rate less than 12 breaths per minute. Medication pushed through patent PIV in L hand then flushed with 10 mL NS. Immediate positive response. Patient able to verbalize full name and DOB. Following naloxone administration, charge nurse stayed with patient while primary RN paged on-call provider to notify about event. Dr. Nitedoc returned page within 2 minutes and came to bedside to assess patient shortly thereafter. IV hydromorphone discontinued. Patient will continue to receive PO oxycodone for pain management. No other new orders at this time.

Example of a Rapid Response/Medical Emergency

At 0405, entered patient room with Smith, RN to answer call bell. Patient stated she needed to use restroom. Patient had not yet been out of bed since PACU recovery from hysterectomy five hours prior. Patient with orders to ambulate TID and permitted to ambulate to bathroom. VS stable until this point, see VS flow sheet. Patient assisted to side of bed with nursing staff and gait belt wrapped around patient's waist and secured. Non-skid socks on both feet. Patient reported slight feeling of dizziness upon sitting up, but reported to nursing staff that the feeling passed after about 20 seconds. After feeling of dizziness passed, patient stood at bedside with assistance of nursing staff. Patient able to stand on her own. Nursing staff provided standby assistance. Patient ambulated safely to toilet. Patient sat safely on toilet. Patient stated that she felt no dizziness, vertigo, or light-headedness. Nursing staff gave patient privacy per request, standing outside bathroom door with door cracked. Approximately 30 seconds later, there was a dull thud inside the bathroom. Opened door to find patient lying on floor. Even chest rise and fall, radial pulses palpable. RN immediately used button on wall to call for Rapid Response Team. RN attempted to arouse patient with no response. Rapid assessment revealed no active bleeding. Unsure if patient's head struck any hard surface as fall was unwitnessed. Rapid response team arrived to patient's side at 0411. Summarized report of patient history relayed to team. Fluid bolus initiated by RRT, set of VS taken with mobile machine. BP 70/40 initially, see Vitals in EMR for all VS assessed. ED physician, Dr. Tromma accompanying RRT stated suspected vasovagal response. At approximately 0420, patient aroused to sternal rub and was able to state her name. Patient could not state current date or current president. CBC and BMP drawn by RRT and sent to lab STAT. BP at 0420 was

79/48. Dr. Tromma verbally ordered transfer to higher level of care. Bed available in step-down unit. Patient transferred to hospital bed with the assistance of three RRT staff, no adverse event during transfer to bed. Patient on bed taken to step-down unit accompanied by one RRT member and primary RN caring for patient. Bedside report given to step-down nurse, Joe Joseph. BP taken in step-down unit was 81/50, see VS in EMR for the rest of the full set of VS taken upon arrival. All of receiving nurse's questions answered.

Example of a Code Blue

At 1017, primary RN caring for patient entered room to administer scheduled Ancef. Patient lying supine in bed. RN tried to arouse patient first by saying name, then by shaking patient's arm. RN at this time observed no apparent chest rise or fall. Palpated for radial pulse for approximately 6 seconds, unable to palpate pulse. RN immediately called for help and hit CODE button wall. Flattened bed, placed back board under patient, and began chest compressions per AHA guidelines. Two additional staff members arrived. Crash cart arrived at bedside at 1020 with Code Team.

Code team at bedside at 1020 with crash cart. Pads placed on patient. 1 mg epinephrine administered at 1021 per verbal order from code team captain, Dr. Tromma, in accordance with ACLS protocol. Compressions continued. 1 mg epinephrine given at 1034. Rhythm checked performed, monitor showed asystole as read by Dr. Tromma. Advanced airway obtained at 1035 with respiratory therapist ventilating patient manually. 1 L bolus of NS rapidly infused into patent 18g IV in right AC via pressure bag. 2 mg naloxone administered at 1036 via IV. Rhythm check. Dr. Tromma announced a shockable rhythm at 1036, 200 J shock delivered and compressions resumed immediately. 2 mg magnesium administered via IV at 1037. Possible differential diagnoses discussed at bedside by Dr. Tromma to include possible PE or dissecting AAA. 50 mEq bicarbonate administered via IV at 1038. An assessment of radial pulses at 1039 indicated ROSC, positive for radial pulses and positive for carotid pulses. Manual ventilation continued and patient transferred to ICU for further treatment at 1040.

*For additional in-depth documentation following a code, default to the policy and procedures of your facility. Most facilities have a CODE template on the crash cart, and many prefer the nurse to transcribe the information from the paper code log to the EMR. The recorder responding the code (which could easily be you!) should fill out the code template with times, actions taken, medications given, VS, and patient response. Then, keep the hard copy of the code template in the patient's chart, unless your facility states otherwise.

If it is not an option to stock the code cart with a recorder template, write times, medications, actions, and patient response on a blank sheet of paper or on the code sheet of my **QuickBrain™ Reusable Nurse Report Notebook** (see back of book).

DISCHARGE OR TRANSFER

Other than Routine End of Shift Handoff

By LENA EMPYEMA | www.zephryco.com

Example of Discharge

Patient with new orders to discharge home. Ensured that discharge note was updated by physician. Discussed discharge with patient. Patient stated his wife is on her way to pick him up. Printed discharge paperwork and provided patient with a copy, reading over important points to patient. RN obtained patient signature on discharge paperwork. All of patient's questions answered at this time. Provided patient with clinic phone number for follow-up questions. Provided patient with belongings bags to pack personal belongings. Belongings cross-checked against intake inventory. No items missing. PIV removed from R AC, tip of catheter intact. Clean gauze and self-adherent dressing applied to site, RN instructed patient to leave dressing in place for 30 minutes before removing dressing and disposing of it. Patient's wife arrived to ward at 1130. Patient transported off ward in wheelchair at 1140 accompanied by ward staff with all personal belongings and discharge paperwork in tow.

Example of a Transfer to Outside Facility

Patient with new orders to transfer to Happy Days Skilled Nursing Facility. Per case manager, room available for patient arrival after 12:00. Patient's family aware of plan of care. Called report to Longturm Kare, RN. Relayed patient status, medical history, current medications, last time meds were administered, amount of assistance required for transfers, social history, and pain management. PIV removed, clean gauze and self-adherent dressing applied to site. BLS ambulance arrival to ward at 1430 to transport patient to Happy Days SNF. Patient transported to stretcher with two staff members assisting and secured with safety belts. Patient transported off ward accompanied by EMTs with all belongings in tow, EMTs with copy of patient chart.

Looking for More Resources?

I have just what you need.

Lena Empyema is now part of Zephry Co. This book is just one of the resources available for understanding how to document nursing care.

The book you just read is specific to narrative notes.

My **comprehensive resource to answer all your questions related to charting** is also available on Amazon.

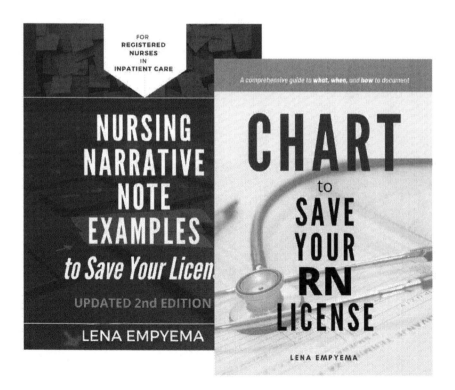

PLUS, my signature tool for inpatient nurses is also in production and available now at www.zephryco.com

Choose my instant-download **Quick & Comprehensive RN Notes & Templates** bundle and copy my working template directly into your EMR.

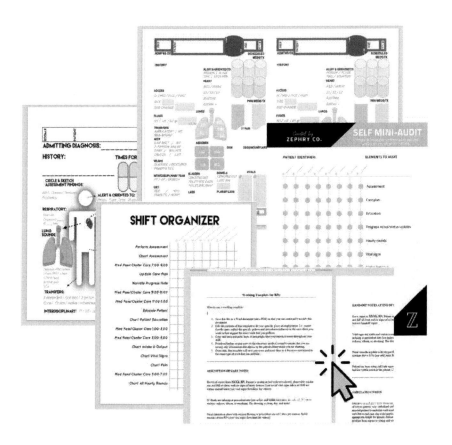

Add on a reusable QuickBrain report notebook to your order and I'll ship it to you for free!

The **ZEPHRY QuickBrain™** is a full color, fully reusable nurse report book that includes mini audit prompts. This report book is a *game changer!*

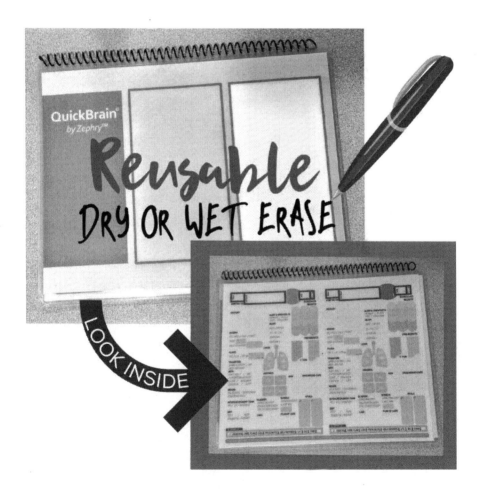

Made in the USA
Middletown, DE
21 May 2024

54653144R00051